3-MINUTE
Abs

3-MINUTE
Abs

ISOLATION
DEFINITION
INTENSITY
FOCUS

KURT
BRUNGARDT

HarperPerennial
A Division of HarperCollins*Publishers*

HarperCollins books may be purchased for educational, business, or sales promotional use. For information please write: Special Markets Department, HarperCollins Publishers, Inc., 10 East 53rd Street, New York, NY 10022.

FIRST EDITION

Designed by Alma Orenstein

Library of Congress Cataloging-in-Publication Data

Brungardt, Kurt, 1964–
    3-minute abs / by Kurt Brungardt. — 1st ed.
      p. cm.
    ISBN 0-06-095270-9
    1. Exercise. 2. Abdomen—Muscles. I. Title.
GV508.B77   1998
613.7'1–dc21   97-51851

01 02 ❖/RRD 10 9

This book is dedicated to my brothers
and to Bryon and Debbie Holmes
for their continued advice and support

And to the ART FARM

CONTENTS

ACKNOWLEDGMENTS

Because part of this book is about myths and misconceptions, I'd like to mention another big one. You never do anything on your own in this world. When I finish a book, this rings most true. And it is something worth hanging on to, even when I'm not working on a project. You never do anything alone in this world.

I would like to thank my brothers and Bryan and Becky Chase for their help. Thank you Raymond Shurtz for helping at crunch time. Special thanks to Mallory Dill who helped line by line while entertaining my dog, Zoe, and me in the process. And, of course, many thanks to photographers Andrew Brucker (cover) and Russ Oliver (exercises).

Also, thanks go out to the usual players who make it all happen: my agent, Dan Strone; my editor, Mauro DiPreta; his assistant, Molly Hennessey; and the whole production team that works so hard, which no one outside the walls of HarperCollins knows about, except the author, who sees how things go in and how they come out.

CHAPTER 1

Common Sense

WHY THE AB OBSESSION?

Abs are the center of your strength and power.
Every time you lift, bend, twist, shift weight,
or balance, you use your abs for both
stabilization and transference of power. Strong
abs are essential for good posture and a
healthy lower back. The abs are also the
center of physical beauty. Someone with a
tight stomach automatically gets a check mark
for having a good body. And the millions of
dollars spent each year on "ab mania"
confirms that everyone wants a trim and
toned midsection. Because abs are the key
to health and beauty, the obsession is
understandable.

THE TRUTH IS SIMPLE

Ernest Hemingway said, "The best reason to tell the truth is because it's the easiest thing to remember." When it comes to abs, it seems like the powers that be don't want us to remember the truth. They surround us with so many misconceptions and myths, so many machines, routines, and miracle diets, that it's nearly impossible to remember a few simple truths.

If something sounds too good to be true, it probably is too good to be true. Perfect abdominals have a history of being pitched like medicine-show miracle cures: girdle belts, plastic sweat suits, and belt machines that jiggle your love handles. And now we have a new generation of contraptions, the most popular being the ab rollers. The irony is you already have the best possible machine to train your abs to perfection—your body. For almost every other body part you need weights or a machine; it would be senseless to train your biceps without weights to curl. But you are born with everything you need to train your abs. You don't need to worry about buying any specialized equipment.

THE THREE KEYS

The truth for the vast majority of us is simple and easy to remember. It contains three key principles. To tone and trim your midsection you have to do three things:

1. Specific exercises for your abs.
2. Consistent aerobic work to burn calories and systematically reduce body fat.
3. A low-calorie, balanced, healthy diet.

EXPECTATIONS

SPOT REDUCING

With so much focus on trimming the abs, the myth of spot reduction has become a mainstream belief. It's as if we've forgotten the physiological fact: **you cannot spot reduce**. The body loses weight systematically and holistically, not one body part at a time. Think of a tennis player. He uses his grip and forearm muscles with greater intensity and frequency in his racquet arm. This makes his racquet arm more muscular than his other arm. But he doesn't have less fat on that arm. He doesn't have one fat arm and one toned arm. You can't lose fat in just your love handles or your lower abs. You will only lose it systematically throughout your entire body.

LIFE ISN'T FAIR

The abs are a natural problem area because we are genetically predisposed to store body fat in our middles. This is called **the first and last principle**. Our middle is the first place we store fat and the last place we take it off. So you can be in really good shape, eat a healthy, smart diet, and still be carrying a little fat around your belly. It's natural.

Yes (I know), this is discouraging in a society that emphasizes a perfect middle. It's just not fair; the one place your body wants to store fat is the one place you most want to get rid of fat.

This makes abs the perfect area to exploit for gimmicks and gadgets. For entrepreneurs, this well never runs dry. It is the problem that will never be solved. This is why the rest of your body can be slim, your face may even become gaunt, and your abs will still have the inch you can pinch. Take heart and know, this little pinch is natural and healthy, and to get rid of it takes extreme and unnatural methods.

UNHEALTHY ICONS

This doesn't mean you can't trim and tone your abs. The important thing is to know what you are up against so you don't get discouraged and give up. Knowing the truth will better prepare you for battle.

In the battle of the abs, we are surrounded by deceptive and damaging media images. Everywhere you look (billboards, movies, and magazines) beautiful bodies abound. It doesn't matter if you're a man or a woman. It could be Calvin Klein underwear ads, Victoria's Secret catalogs, *International Male,* or any fitness or fashion magazine. You can't help being affected. You see these images over and over and at an unconscious level you literally become addicted to beauty. But these images are not the truth. They are fantasy created to sell products. The photographers shoot at the most flattering angles; they use light and shadow to accent the beautiful and hide the flaws. And they airbrush away any remaining imperfections to create their carefully manipulated sculpture.

On top of this, the models go through extreme and unhealthy measures to achieve their look. They often starve and dehydrate before a shoot. Plus, they have more time to work out. Staying in shape is their job. And if this is not enough, when the camera clicks the models are flexing and sucking in their abs. They may be smiling and looking casual, but believe me, down below they're flexing and sucking. A model can learn to cover up many flaws by mastering posing techniques. That's why they get paid the big bucks. The truth is, Mr. Olympia and supermodels don't look in picture-peak condition 365 days a year.

BE A REALIST/BE A DREAMER

Approaching abs truthfully means being a realist, an optimistic and positive realist. Being a realist isn't always easy, because it often means letting go of your fantasies. Knowing the facts, however, prepares you to reach your potential. Unrealistic expectations ultimately leave you disillusioned and discouraged because you never reach your goal. And believing the marketing claims of the product of the month leaves you feeling like a loser because you can't live up to the promises (false claims), and you quit. The marketplace loves this. It means you'll soon be shopping for another miracle product, hoping your fantasy can come true.

Don't misunderstand, you need a dream. A dream is an essential part of motivation. It drives you forward. It's what makes you human. But you don't need a dream that's guaranteed to turn into a nightmare. What you have to do is a paradox: Be a realist and be a dreamer. Know the facts about training, know your body type, and dream about creating the perfect you, fulfilling 100 percent of your potential.

WHAT TO EXPECT

Ab training can be discouraging because it is hard to see quick results. You train and train, but your stomach looks the same. Other body parts are different. When you work your biceps, you see the muscle get pumped in the mirror, and after a few weeks you are flexing for your friends. Because we carry a little extra fat around our middles, we can't see the muscles work when we exercise. And since this is the last area where the weight goes off, we don't see quick results. But if you stay with this routine, your abs will grow stronger and firmer underneath. And if you faithfully do your cardiovascular work and eat smart, slowly but surely your body fat will decrease and those new, shapely abs will emerge.

REMEMBER

- Don't expect to have ultrachiseled abs year round.
- Don't expect to totally rid yourself of that little extra inch of flesh around your love handles and lower abs, unless you're prepared to go through extreme measures like a professional bodybuilder does.
- Be consistent using the three keys. There is not a quick and easy way to achieve great abs.
- Be patient and keep the *first and last principle* in mind; know what is natural and healthy for the body.
- Don't be a victim of media icons; call on the power of the truth.
- Set realistic goals, dreaming of your best self.
- Enjoy the process and the health benefits along the way.
    Healthier lower back.
    Better posture.
    More enjoyment and better performance in recreational activities (the abs are essential for stability, balance, and transference of movements in virtually all activities).

The 3-Minute Revolution

CHAPTER 2

THE PARADOX

What people want from a workout program is a paradox. They want to invest a minimum amount of time and get maximum results. This desire is what leaves people open to gimmicks and gadgets. Pondering a way to bridge this paradox and create an ab program based on sound training principles yet requiring a minimum amount of time was the motivation for this book. You train your abs just three minutes in each workout session.

For any exercise program to be effective you need to do it consistently. As intimidating as it may sound, exercise is a lifetime commitment. *3-Minute Abs* is a training system you can stick with. It does no good to work out one month and then take the next month off.

3-Minute Abs allows fitness to become part of your lifestyle, without changing your lifestyle.

ABDOMINAL DELINQUENTS

Abs are the body's problem child. They just don't seem to respond to training like other muscles. *3-Minute Abs* is the answer for this rebel body part.

The reason your abs don't respond like other muscles is simple. *You haven't trained them like other muscles.* For the first time, a program brings FOUR KEY training principles to ab work.

THE FOUR PRINCIPLES

- Body Area Isolation
- Rest/Recuperation
- Intensity
- Focus

Bodybuilders and professional athletes have been applying these principles to other muscle groups (with great results) for years. But no one has used all these proven principles to create an abdominal program.

THE 3-MINUTE REVOLUTION
How the Four Principles Work

PRINCIPLE 1: BODY AREA ISOLATION

Bodybuilders have always broken down their workouts into separate body parts: leg day, chest and back day, shoulders and arms day, etc. This way each body part gets an intense and focused workout. And most importantly, on a three-day rotation, each part gets plenty of recuperation time for strengthening and sculpting each area.

But most people train their entire abdominal area in a single workout session. This takes a large chunk of time and becomes monotonous. The downward spiral is predictable: Your workouts lose intensity, you stop seeing and feeling the benefits, and then you quit exercising. It's not a character flaw. It's your program.

3-Minute Abs separates your abdominal training into three parts, avoiding all these pitfalls and allowing you to train with greater intensity while avoiding burnout.

> ### THE *3-MINUTE AB* ROUTINE
>
> - Day one: Lower abs
> - Day two: Obliques
> - Day three: Upper abs
>
> *Take a day off and start the rotation over again.

PRINCIPLE 2: RECUPERATION

Exercising just one area in a workout session solves one of the biggest ab training dilemmas. *How often do I train my abs? Can I train them every day? Or are they like every other muscle?* There is no simple answer to these questions. The abs are like other muscles and yet they are a special case.

A muscle's makeup is determined by its function. The abs are posture muscles; in other words, they help hold you up all day. Because of this function, they consist primarily of slow-twitch fibers (endurance fibers), which recover faster and can be trained more often. This makes your abs different from other muscles, which consist of primarily fast-twitch fibers (explosive), meaning they tire faster and need more time to recover.

The muscle's composition helps answer the "how often" dilemma. Because abs are slow twitch (recover faster), you can train them more frequently than other muscle groups, but you don't need to train them every day.

3-Minute Abs solves this problem. You train three days in a row, hitting each area with maximum intensity while at the same time giving each area maximum rest. And on an area's rest days, the muscle functions as a helper, getting a light, toning workout. This is a prescription for success.

PRINCIPLE 3: INTENSITY

Intensity is the most important training principle in terms of achieving your goals. Technically, intensity means how you overload the muscle to stimulate development. In practical terms, it means how hard you work. Working just one ab area a day is the most effective way to overload your abdominal muscles for peak results. That's why bodybuilders train one or two body parts a day. To get the optimum benefits from training you have to push yourself to muscular failure. No one likes to go to this point of pain.

3-Minute Abs only asks you to go to muscular failure once per workout. A traditional routine requires you to go through the pain three times (once for each ab area). You probably zone out at the two- or three-minute mark in your ab workout anyway. Everything after that point is a waste. It's hard to push yourself for eight or more minutes. *3-Minute Abs* gives you a structure that fosters an intense workout, creating a routine that puts you in the zone, not a routine that causes you to zone out.

PRINCIPLE 4: FOCUS

Focus is your ability to keep your eye on the prize, in the short term and the long term. In the short term, it means concentrating on the muscle you are working. Because your workout is only three minutes, it is easy to commit to this focus. There's less of a chance for your mind to start planning dinner in the middle of your routine. In the long term, it is easier to stay motivated because you see the same ab area and the same set of exercises once every four days. This keeps the routines fresh.

WHY *3-MINUTE ABS* WORKS

- It enables you to train your abs with greater intensity.
- It gives each area maximum recuperation.
- It reduces burnout factor.
- It creates a strong mind-body focus.
- Different routines create variety.
- It takes just three minutes.

We can all find three minutes: in the morning, before lunch or dinner, after work, during a commercial break, before you go to bed, etc. The single most important exercise factor is consistency over time. This is a program you can stick with, which means you'll see results. *3-Minute Abs* will give you what you really want: a simple routine based on advanced training principles and the best possible results with a minimum investment of time.

3-Minute Anatomy

3-MINUTE ANATOMY LESSON

You don't have to be an expert in anatomy to trim and tone your midsection, but knowing the basics will help you visualize the muscles you are training. This chapter will explain and illustrate the three primary muscles you will be training.

RECTUS ABDOMINIS

The rectus abdominis is the large sheath of muscle that runs from your pubic bone to your sternum. This is the muscle people are talking about when they refer to the abs as a "six-pack" or use the term *washboard abs*.

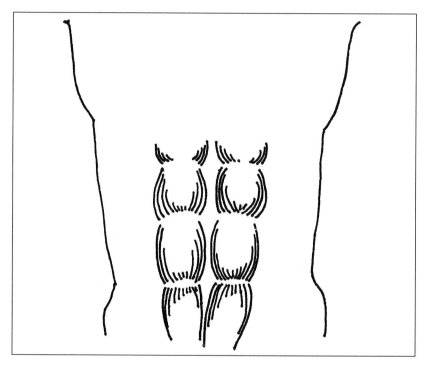

Illustration of Rectus Abdominis

THE OBLIQUES: EXTERNAL AND INTERNAL

The obliques run from the front half of the hip and the crest of the pubic bone to the ribs (just below the chest). The obliques also attach to the rectus abdominis and the seratus muscle (the muscle that covers the ribs). These muscles are commonly known as the love handles. They frame and highlight the rectus and cut the shape of the torso as it rises from the hips to the chest.

The obliques run diagonally to the rectus abdominis as shown in the photos below. The external and internal obliques crisscross each other, creating a web effect.

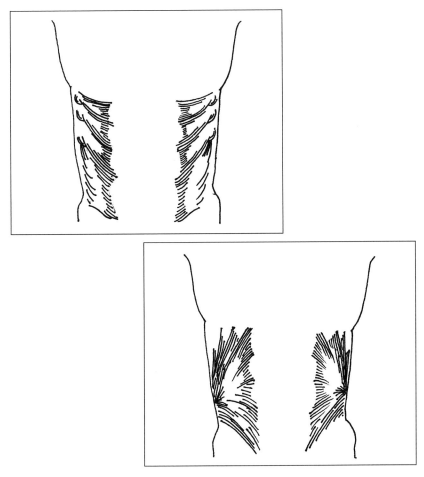

Illustration of External Obliques and Internal Obliques (as its name suggests, the external oblique lies on top of the internal oblique in this web).

CHAPTER 4

3-Minute Kinesiology

BASIC KINESIOLOGY

Kinesiology is the study of how your body moves: which muscles contract and move specific parts of your body. You need to understand a few basic principles to always be in touch with the ab area you're training.

UPPER ABS

The easiest place to start is with the upper abs, because most of us are familiar with the basic crunch.

Two basic things are happening when you crunch: (1) your shoulder blades are coming off the mat, and (2) your rib cage is moving toward your hips. So, as a rule of thumb:

Anytime your rib cage is moving toward your hips in an ab area, you are emphasizing your upper abdominal.

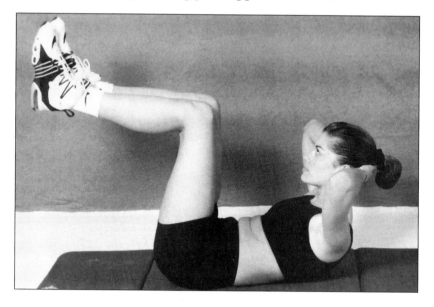

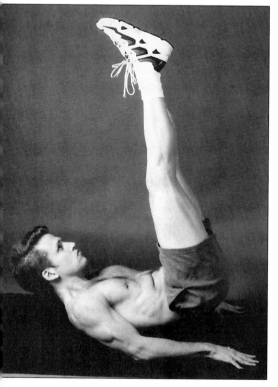

LOWER ABS

When you work the lower abs, you do the opposite. A good example of this is the reverse crunch.

Again, two basic things are happening when you do a reverse crunch: (1) your hips come off the mat, and (2) your hips move toward your rib cage. Another rule of thumb: **Anytime your hips move toward your rib cage in an ab exercise, you are emphasizing your lower abdominal**.

OBLIQUES

You are training your obliques whenever you execute a twisting or crossing motion with your torso. A crossover crunch is a good example of this motion.

Again, two basic things are happening when you do a crossover crunch: (1) one shoulder blade comes off the mat, and (2) one side of your rib cage moves toward the opposite side of your hip. So, as a rule of thumb: **Anytime one side of your rib cage crosses or twists toward the opposite side of your hip, you are emphasizing your obliques**.

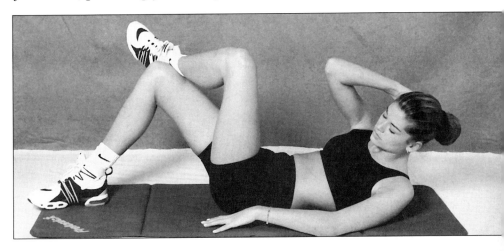

You are also working your obliques whenever you move your rib cage directly toward the side of your hip. An easy illustration of this is a side bend.

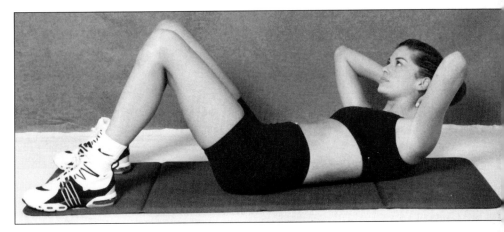

These simple movement guidelines will allow you to analyze any abdominal movement and determine which area or combination of areas an ab exercise is emphasizing.

CHAPTER 5

Using Your Body

GOOD TRAINING HABITS

The next two chapters cover good training habits for the body and mind. You need to know the basics for two simple reasons:

1. So you can get the best results in the least amount of time.
2. So you can exercise injury free.

Even though this book focuses on abs, establishing good training habits means eventually incorporating the FOUR FITNESS ELEMENTS into your total program. The four fitness elements are: strength training, cardiovascular training, a stretching program, and a healthy diet. There will be more on this later.

THE NECK AND THE HEAD

Two important areas to focus on when training your abs are the neck and lower back support. Let's start with the neck.

With the invention of ab rollers, neck strain and comfort have become a prominent concern. It is important that you do not experience significant neck pain. It is also easy to achieve this comfort without a special machine. I would venture to say that it's easier using just your body.

Your neck may hurt when you do sit-ups, but the neck isn't the culprit. The problem is your big old head that weighs around ten pounds. To get rid of neck pain, you have to focus on the head.

Technique: There are two main rules you should keep in mind to prevent neck strain:

1. RULE ONE: When doing ab work you should always try to maintain a space about the size of an apple (or your fist) between your chin and chest.

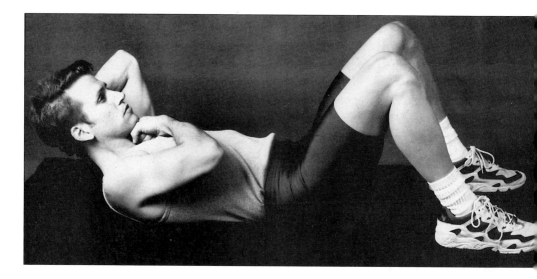

2. RULE TWO: Support your head to maintain this position. The easiest ways to do this are with your hands or a towel.

Using a Towel (opposite)

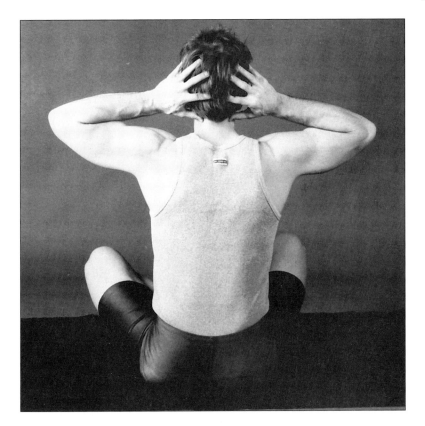

The Hands: The best way to ease the stress on your neck for basic crunch movements is to support your head with your fingertips.

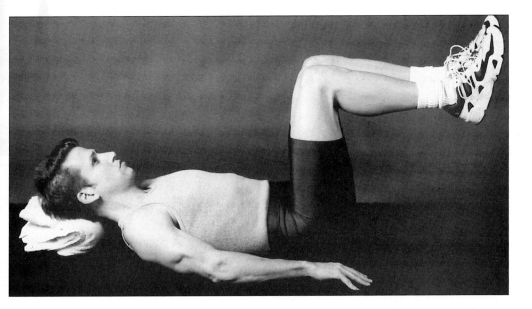

Notice the hand position in the photo: The fingers are spread wide, the thumbs are placed at the top of the neck, and the pinkie is at the top of the head, building a bridge between your neck and head.

This takes the stress off your neck.

In this position your hands, arms, and shoulders are doing the work, not the neck. But you have to make a mental shift to allow the head to relax, letting the hands, arms, and shoulders take over. We are conditioned to use our neck to hold up the head. This is natural. So you have to give your neck muscles the message, "Let go." It takes a little practice. But if you keep giving the neck the message, it will quickly start to trust your hands, arms, and shoulders to do the work, and your neck strain will disappear.

The ab rollers present the same problem. Even though there's a pad to rest your head on, you will unconsciously hold with the neck unless you "let go."

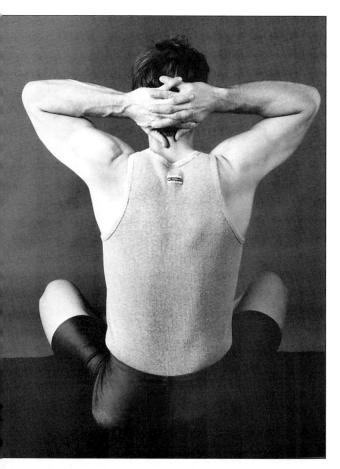

Common Mistakes:

A common mistake is to interlace your fingers behind your head and pull on the head as you crunch. This breaks rule one, driving the chin toward the chest, creating stress.

ONE-HAND METHOD

This technique leaves the other hand free to feel the ab area you are working. Again, the key to this method is building the bridge. Spread your thumbs and pinkies wide (thumb at the top of your neck, fingers spread across the head). Having a free hand to place on the working muscle helps create the mind-muscle link. More on this in the next chapter.

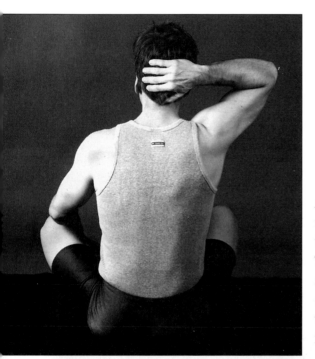

Another simple technique is using a towel to support the head. To get the best results, spread the towel out, creating a wide web with the area supporting your head.

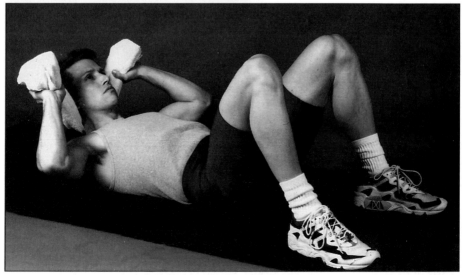

PROPER STARTING POSITION: READY, SET, GO

Proper starting position is a place of READINESS: Your back is neither arched nor rounded, and your pelvis is slightly tilted (accomplished by gently squeezing your buttocks together). This causes your lower back to press against the floor and your belly button to move down toward your spine. Consciously lock yourself in this position before you start your set.

READINESS also means creating the right MIND-SET, the right attitude. You need to bring your mind to a point of concentration and focus (more on this in the next chapter). Ready the body, set the mind, and GO.

THE BASIC PRINCIPLES

WARMING UP

It is always important to warm your body up before exercising. Warming up prepares the body for action.

1. It increases blood flow in the muscles, making the muscles more efficient.
2. It increases muscle temperature, allowing the muscles to contract more forcefully and with more speed.
3. It reduces injury potential.

Ideally, you should warm up your body with five minutes of light aerobic work before training your abs. You may also find it helpful to stretch key areas like your neck and lower back (see pages 63 to 67).

STARTING OUT

One of the most frequently asked questions is, "How much should I do when I start my program?" In this book, you have a specific routine, but everyone will start this process from a different point.

In the beginning focus on mastering the technique. The fastest way to learn a new technique is to practice it when you are fresh. When you have a breakdown in technique, stop and rest. Be patient; don't try to push yourself in the early stages. Once the movements become second nature, you can start to push yourself. Go one step at a time and establish good habits. You're in this for the long haul.

FULL RANGE OF MOTION AND CONSTANT TENSION

It is important to keep resistance on the muscles throughout the entire exercise. Simply stated, during a movement you must maintain constant tension on the muscle, feeling its contraction throughout the full range of motion. Do not let momentum take over. Keep the motion controlled, feeling the muscles do the work.

SPEED OF MOVEMENT

As a rule of thumb, the speed of movement should be slow and controlled for both positive (eccentric) and negative (concentric) contractions.

As you reach advanced levels of training, it is beneficial to vary the speed of movement in order to shock the muscles and add variety to your workouts.

BREATHING

It is important to breathe during ab work. It sounds obvious. But you would be surprised how many people hold their breath when they train.

THE TECHNIQUE

EXHALE through your mouth as you exert effort. In a crunch you exhale as you raise your shoulder blades off the mat.

INHALE through your nose as you release the effort. In a crunch you would inhale as you lower your body back toward the mat.

QUALITY OF THE REP

The most important element in training is not quantity but quality. Don't worry about how many reps you are doing. Concentrate on keeping your technique strict and going through a full range of motion on each repetition. Feel the contraction of each rep; keep constant tension on the ab muscles throughout the movement. Indulge in each and every repetition.

PUSHING FOR AND THROUGH GOOD PAIN

It is also important to know the difference between good pain and bad pain. To have the most effective workout possible, you must exercise through the good pain. Overcoming the obstacle of added repetition and weight causes the muscles to adapt and get stronger. This is difficult because it is not a comfortable experience.

You must fatigue the muscle to get maximum results. The intensity level of your training depends on several variables:

- Your goals.
- Your present state of physical health.
- What your body is telling you on that particular day.

Ideally, you want to be able to push yourself into good pain on every exercise, without forfeiting proper technique. This requires mental toughness; you continue to exercise even though you are experiencing fatigue. This is often referred to as pushing to the pump (good pain). Your mind will try to stop you before this point. You need to learn your limits. And you need to learn to push your limits.

Good Pain: Is the feeling of being pumped, having the muscle fill with blood. And yes, even that burning sensation that comes from lactic acid buildup is a good pain. These are feelings you will eventually thrive on. Pushing past your normal limits is part of the satisfaction that comes from working out. In the beginning it may just feel like pain. But one day it will be pleasure.

Bad Pain: Is a warning sign. It means you've injured yourself.

When you feel this type of pain, stop immediately. If you have lower-back problems, be aware of your lower back at all times. Warning signs are shooting pains, sharp pains, and spasms. Whenever pain moves out of the area you're working, it is a good idea to stop and evaluate. Don't push through bad pain.

SORENESS

Muscle soreness is common after a workout. Don't worry if you're a little sore (good pain). Soreness is a result of microscopic tears in muscle tissue. They need recuperation time to repair. If you are too sore to train during your next session, you have overdone it. Most of the time it is good to train through soreness. The increased blood flow and movement in the area will help repair the tissue.

TRAINING TIPS FOR AB ROLLERS

The following is a list of guidelines to help you get the most out of training with an ab roller. It is important to remember that you are still responsible for the integrity of the movement. The machine doesn't magically solve all the problems and do all the work for you. It creates a new set of problems. This shouldn't discourage you, but you need to be aware of the obstacles and have techniques to solve them. The danger with the ab roller is the misconception that all you have to do is get in it and rock and roll. You are still responsible for the exercise. And the fact that you are adjusting to a machine, which can't give you detailed feedback like your body, makes these obstacles more difficult.

1. Make sure the neck pad does not slide down from your head to your neck when you execute your crunch. You have to adjust your head with the roller as you go through the exercise's range of motion. The neck pad has a tendency to push your chin to your chest. This has the same effect as pulling your neck forward with your hands (as in the previous photo).
2. Don't push the roller down with your elbows.

3. Don't push the roller down with your hands or squeeze the roller tightly with your hands.
4. Make sure the entire unit doesn't creep forward.
5. Let your neck relax into the pad.
6. You control the roller; don't let the roller control you. In other words, don't let momentum take over. You need to control both the upward and downward phases of the movement.

CHAPTER 6

Using Your Mind

THE MIND

One of the key factors in achieving peak results has nothing to do with ab rollers, proper technique, or diets. It has to do with harnessing the power of your mind.

Integration of mind and body has become a popular topic. Their interdependency is well documented as a crucial link for both physical and mental health. A mind programmed for failure will inevitably fail. The information you give your subconscious, the images you feed it, will play a big role in determining the result of any endeavor. Sportscasters describe this state as being in a zone. In recent years sports psychology has developed techniques that help professional and Olympic athletes train their minds just as they train their bodies.

The techniques that work for them will also help you improve. This section will discuss and teach you the basic skills of relaxation, concentration, visualization, and power phrases.

Good mental habits mean more than just going through the motions. A good workout is a combination of body (technique) and mind (focus). In the long run, the hardest habits to establish are mental. The mind is much more of a trickster than the body.

In our daily lives our focus is weak and drifts, as if it were out of our control. In our culture, this drifting is associated with our inalienable right to freedom: I can think whatever I want whenever I want. Our culture (mass media and advertising) promotes distraction and disassociation. Our minds really aren't free. They drift and jump from place to place instead of focusing in the moment on the task at hand.

Focus and concentration are powerful. They allow you to see what is really going on. They allow you to tune in and create the moment instead of just letting it passively drift over you. This means you can bring about change. And since we're talking about exercise (aren't we?), this means if you focus, you can change your body. You can start a revolution in your body and bring about real change instead of just going through the motions and then becoming dissatisfied with the results.

That's why athletes and coaches always say the mind separates the best from the rest. At a professional level all the athletes are physically blessed; only those with the mental edge become the best. This edge allows you to achieve your full potential. That is why those who can focus and concentrate are paid the big bucks and why athletes make millions. They're not daydreaming on the court, in practice, or in the weight room. It's the same in corporations; the high salaries go to the leaders who stay focused and solve problems. These leaders and athletes have the freedom to focus their minds when they choose to.

The following techniques will help you train your mind to have freedom of choice (focus when you want, drift when you want) so you can help your body reach its full potential.

THE MIND-MUSCLE LINK

If you believe that the mind and the body must work together to achieve peak performance, then you have to put your mind in the muscle you're training. This metaphorical action puts 100 percent of your focus on the muscle you are training. Body-builders are particularly adept at this technique. This is one of the reasons why they get such spectacular results, while other people work out and complain that they don't see a difference.

THE TECHNIQUE

When you exercise you need to concentrate on the exact muscle you are training. If you are working your lower abs, feel those muscles move your hips back toward your rib cage. You have to indulge in the feeling, the burn, and the fatigue of the muscles as they work. And you need to have an ideal image of that area in your mind's eye. You need to feel and see the muscle move through its full range of motion during each repetition. Every repetition must be filled with this level of quality.

RELAXATION

Relaxation clears the mind and releases tension from the body. It opens up the mind to the suggestions made in the visualization. You will learn two basic relaxation skills in this section: controlled breathing and progressive relaxation.

CONTROLLED BREATHING

One way to achieve a relaxed state is by concentrating on your breathing. Settle in a comfortable position lying down or sitting, and focus on inhaling and exhaling for approximately a minute. Then start to inhale on a count of five and exhale on a count of five, until you feel that your breathing pattern is smooth and regular.

Next focus on feeling the air coming into your lungs and imagine it being transported to every cell of your body. Every time you breathe out, let any negative thoughts or feelings you might have leave your body with the breath. And each time you breathe in, imagine the breathe purifying and energizing your body. If it helps, imagine the breath entering your body as a white cleansing light. Continue this process until you feel a release of muscular tension and a feeling of being centered. Now you are ready for visualization and positive suggestions.

PROGRESSIVE RELAXATION

Another way to prepare for visualization and positive programming is to consciously relax from your toes to your head.

Settle in a comfortable position, either lying or sitting, and take a couple of deep breaths. Give your body the message to relax. Then start to feel where your body is making contact with the floor or the chair. If you're lying down, feel your heels, buttocks, shoulders, and head touching the floor. Then move your focus down to your feet. Send the message to relax, telling all the little muscles on the soles of your feet and across the top of your feet to let go. Move up to your calves, and give them the message to relax. Move up to your thighs and hamstrings, telling them to relax. Go to the muscles of your buttocks and tell them to relax. Then move to your lower back, middle back, and upper back, giving your entire back the message to relax. Send the message to your shoulders, arms, hands, chest, and stomach, telling them to relax. And finish with your neck, head, face, and throat. Tell all the little muscles around your eyes, cheeks, and jaws to relax. Tell your forehead and scalp to relax. After you have given your entire body, part by part, the message to relax, allow yourself to go deeper and deeper into relaxation with each breath, giving in to gravity and melting into the floor.

When you have reached a desired level of relaxation, you are ready for visualization and positive programming.

To bring yourself out of this state, simply say, "On a count of three I will open my eyes, feeling relaxed and with a reserve of energy, ready to go on with my day." This technique is also good to do with a partner; have him or her take you through the process.

VISUALIZATION

THE PSYCHOLOGY OF VISUALIZATION

You are what you perceive yourself to be. Throughout life

your experiences have shaped the way you view yourself. Every success and every failure has an impact on your identity, confidence, and chances for future success. Because we all learn by trial and error, we all tend to have more failures than successes. It starts at birth and continues through childhood and on into adolescence. The very nature of these life phases (dependence on others, having to obey parents and teachers) reinforces the belief that people will always be bigger, stronger, wiser, and above all will possess more power than you.

As an adult, these negative thoughts, feelings, and experiences continue to have a powerful impact on how you act, react, and feel about yourself. These early messages can also affect how high you set your goals and how willing you are to achieve them.

Visualization can be an effective method for reversing the negative beliefs that stem from your past experiences. Visualization allows you to overwhelm those past negative messages with a steady input of positive images. The brain is like a computer. It behaves exactly the way it has been programmed. The only way to erase a bad program is to reprogram a better one. You can overcome your past failures by programming for future success.

Many of the world's greatest athletes have used visualization successfully for years. In fact, athletes were visualizing long before anyone gave it a name. Jack Nicklaus always previews his golf shot mentally before ever beginning the swing. Divers, dancers, and gymnasts all know the value of practicing mentally before performing. Most successful athletes use some form of visualization to help them perform better, as do most successful businesspeople. In fact, successful people in all walks of life usually include some form of visualization among their techniques for achieving their goals. We all do it when we dream of the future: a new car, a big house in the country, kids, etc. As you train yourself to imagine success, you cease to concentrate on failure.

VISUALIZATION BASICS

In a nutshell, visualization is the creation of mental pictures. At an unconscious level you are constantly creating images. These pictures program your self-image. The goal of visualization is to consciously create positive images to help you achieve the goals you want.

To achieve the abs you want, you must be able to see them in your mind's eye. Your image could be a picture from a magazine, the way you looked a few years ago, someone you saw on the beach, or any combination of these things. What's important is that you create a specific image of how you want your abs to look. It is important to keep an element of truth and realism in your picture. Create an image that fits your genetic type and potential, a picture you can believe in with every cell of your body, not one that is impossible. Your picture can change and evolve and refine itself. You are not locked into one image forever.

The more vivid the visualization, the more effective it will be. It is essential to use sensory details. Imagine how defined your abs will be. See the separation of the muscles. See the color of your skin. See the washboard layering of your muscles. What do they feel like to touch? Make the snapshot of your ideal abs as clear as possible.

Imagine how these new abs make you feel physically and emotionally. Feel their tightness, the hardness of the muscles. See how others react to them. Walk down the beach with them. See your lover's response.

To be effective you must visualize every day (or night), not just when you feel like it. Any negative aspects existing in the subconscious took years to formulate and will not disappear overnight. However, with a consistent visualization strategy, you can begin to change these negative aspects and program for success.

PROGRAMMING POWER PHRASES

Power programming is the creation of an affirmation phrase that will help push you to achieve your goals. These phrases don't have to be detailed. But they must be evocative enough to eliminate negative thoughts. Phrases such as "I'm the man!" or "You go, girl!" are examples of power phrases. Get in the habit of using them extensively, especially when you feel doubts or negative thoughts creeping into your mind. Everyone experiences these doubts. People who succeed fight through their doubts, no matter how extreme they may be. Every person has the ability to overcome these negative thoughts and doubts, but many people give in to them. With the application of these two techniques your chances of overcoming this negative programming will be greatly improved.

PLANNING YOUR SUCCESS

We want everything: a perfect body, a challenging job, a great love life, and time for recreation and entertainment. How do you manage all these wants in a twenty-four-hour time period? You have to make choices and prioritize your needs. If you had the time you might spend two hours a day in the gym. But you don't have the time. So you need to be honest with yourself and figure out how much time you can spend each week training your body. After you've made that choice, don't feel guilty about it. **With your fitness goals it is much better to err on the side of doing a little less, but doing it consistently, than trying to do too much and quitting.** The key is to be honest with yourself and set realistic goals.

After you have set your goal, the next step is owning it. This means writing it down. Remember, a goal is not a goal unless it is written down. Then read your goals every day. It does no good to write them down if you don't read them. Read them on days when you're excited about working out; read them on days when you're not. Say them out loud, take responsibility for them.

When making goals you will find the following format useful. You should create long-term, intermediate, and short-term goals and daily tasks.

Long-Term Goals: Write down where you would like to be a year from now. Be specific. For example: You want washboard abs. You might have a picture from a magazine of how you want to look. Cut it out and paste it next to the written goal.

Intermediate Goals: Write down where you want to be in six months. If you consistently work your abs for six months, you can accomplish some very noticeable improvements.

Short-Term Goals: Write down where you want to be a month from now. Every month you need to update this goal, always keeping in mind the results you want in six months and in a year. Examples might be:

- Losing a certain amount of weight or body fat.
- Establishing a consistent workout schedule.
- Developing a certain amount of strength and endurance by lifting two to three times a week.

Daily Tasks: At the beginning of each day set at least two goals for that day. You can also do this planning at night before you go to bed. Write them down.

Be specific. You should include not only what the task is but also at what time it will be performed. For example, on Monday your daily tasks might be: (1) ab workout (specific program) at 8:00 A.M., and (2) salad and a whole-wheat roll for lunch.

Setting goals is one thing, following through is another. You need to be patient and keep the fire burning. You need to get motivated and stay motivated.

MOTIVATION

Motivation is the primary reason people hire personal trainers. They don't think they can do it themselves. This book is designed to act as your personal trainer, giving you a clear program that you can do by yourself.

Motivation is also a very personal thing. There are hundreds of motivational tapes and books and a cable TV system filled with infomercial gurus. The bottom line is, do what works for you. Ultimately, motivation has to come from deep within. No one can just give it to you. Otherwise it doesn't have any power.

So take your motivation wherever you can get it. Cut out photos from magazines, let sports heroes like Michael Jordan inspire you, let old lovers push you to the next level, let anger inspire you (work it right out of your body), schedule a vacation on the beach, or just enjoy working out because it feels good.

You need to continually find new ways to motivate yourself. Because with your training there are no shortcuts. And you have to be consistent. That means you're in it for the long haul. Love the struggle.

CHAPTER 7

Introduction to the Program

3-Minute Abs sounds easy. Don't be fooled. It's an *intense* three minutes. In sports terms it equals a round of boxing, a period in Olympic wrestling, and approximately the time it takes an elite runner to finish a mile race. Like I said, there is no easy way to achieve trimmed and defined abdominals. So as you start the program, don't be discouraged if you can't do each three-minute routine without resting. Listen to know your body and progress at your own pace.

HOW TO USE THIS BOOK

FOLLOWING THE PLAN

The program is easy to follow. You train your abs three days, take a day off, then start the rotation again. Each routine will have specific instructions, showing you step by step how to complete that day's routine. The overall program goes like this: DAY ONE, you train your lower abs; DAY TWO, you train your obliques; DAY THREE, you train your upper abs.

FLEXIBILITY

Because schedules change and life has a way of getting chaotic, the system becomes flexible by simply combining days. But don't get in the habit of doing this.

Combining days means doing two workouts in one session. This would translate into six-minute abs. For example, let's say DAY ONE lands on Monday and you have an incredibly busy day at work, dinner, and a date. You probably aren't going to do your abs in front of your date. So on Tuesday you combine DAY ONE and TWO in a workout.

Or let's say it's a Thursday and you're on DAY TWO. And you know tomorrow (Friday) you won't have time to work out. So you plan ahead and combine DAY TWO and THREE on Thursday, because you don't want to be on your date thinking, "Gee, my upper abs feel a little flabby."

But remember, it only takes three minutes. That's the beauty of the program. You can even do it on the busiest days (in the morning, at night before you hop in the shower, etc.). So don't fall into lazy habits.

MAINTENANCE PERIODS

Sometimes life gets so hectic that it's hard to find even three minutes. Or you feel burned out and need to ease off a little bit. Instead of coming to a complete stop you can transition into a maintenance program. The goal of a maintenance period is to maintain the benefits you've worked to achieve. On a mainte-nance program, follow the same rotation, but just do one rotation a week. This would mean that in a seven-day period you would train three days and take four off.

Another way to handle a maintenance phase is to choose one exercise from each routine, creating a single three-minute routine that works all three areas. You should do this routine two to three times a week. Remember, during a maintenance phase, the results you've worked for will eventually start to fade.

WEIGHT RESISTANCE

You can add weight resistance on almost any ab exercise. This is normally done with the use of weight plates, dumbbells, ankle weights, or a medicine ball. You should add light weights if the routine becomes too easy. Adding weight increases the intensity. The safest way to add weight for upper abs and obliques is to place a weight across your chest.

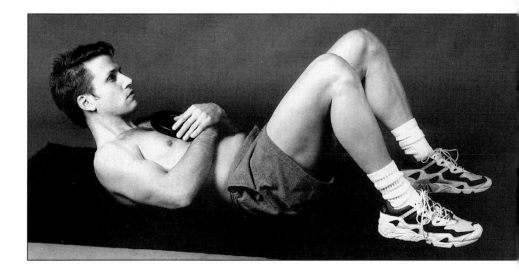

The safest way to add weight for lower-ab exercises is to place a dumbbell between your feet or between your knees.

When adding resistance, you may find ankle weights the most comfortable for lower-ab movements.

Another way to add resistance is to do these exercises on a slant board.

TRAINER'S TIPS

The following tips are essential for ab work:

- Keep constant tension on the abs.
- Keep motion slow and controlled, no bouncing or jerking.
- Pause for a contraction at the top of the movement.
- Don't rest at the beginning of each repetition before going on to the next one. Let your shoulder blades or hips just lightly touch the floor. Don't give your body weight to the floor.
- When possible, keep locked in your position of readiness: slight pelvic tilt, belly button lowered toward the spine.
- Focus your mind on feeling your abs do the work, putting your mind in the muscle. Place a hand on the working area to help create the link. Don't just go through the motions.
- Let your head relax into your hand(s) or a towel, taking stress off your neck.

KNOW THYSELF

This means know your fitness level: Are you a beginner, an intermediate, or an advanced exerciser? The following section outlines these three levels and gives you some simple guidelines for taking the next step.

BEGINNING LEVEL

If you are a first-time exerciser or if you have taken an extended break from training, you will probably not be able to complete the routine using proper technique. During each session you will need to stop and rest, starting again when you're ready. Even if you are resting, it is important to stay within the three-minute time frame. Do what you can in three minutes. Your strength and endurance will gradually increase.

If you are just starting out, don't push yourself too hard in the beginning. This can lead to excessive soreness. Patience and consistency are the key virtues at this stage of the game.

Guidelines:

1. When learning a new movement, practice it while you are fresh. In other words, not when you're exhausted at the end

of a workout or late at night. This can lead to unnecessary frustration.

2. In the beginning, your main focus should be on mastering proper technique. Focus on technique until you can do the movement correctly without thinking, even when you are tired.

3. Try to gradually add another FITNESS ELEMENT (strength training, cardio/aerobic work, stretching, nutrition) to your program.

INTERMEDIATE LEVEL

If you fall into the intermediate level, this is probably not the first fitness book you've purchased. You most likely buy or look through fitness magazines. And you probably own videotapes and/or a piece of home-fitness equipment. These are all positive things. On the negative side, you probably suffer from the start-and-stop syndrome, sometimes for extended periods of time (falling out of your program for a month or more). Trying to keep in shape and eat right have been goals you've struggled to integrate into your life for at least two years. Also, you attempt to include at least two FITNESS ELEMENTS in your workout.

Guidelines:

1. At this level you need to start pushing yourself, increasing your intensity. Indulge in the feelings of good pain (page 26).

2. Consistency, consistency, consistency. This is the level where most exercisers get stuck. *3-Minute Abs* is designed to help you stay consistent and move to the next level.

3. Make a commitment to up the stakes. Either increase your training in a FITNESS ELEMENT or add another FITNESS ELEMENT to your workout. For example:

    Add five minutes to your cardiovascular training.

    Take an extra class per week.

    If strength training is not part of your program, add weight training to your workout.

THE ADVANCED LEVEL

If you fall into this level, fitness is an important and integral part of your lifestyle and has been for at least two years. Commitment and consistency are not problems. But you tend to be too hard on yourself and overtrain.

Even at this level, you will find *3-Minute Abs* a challenge. Its uniqueness may be just the thing you need to shock your muscles into peak shape.

Guidelines:

1. At this level your challenge is to harness the power of the mind (the mind-muscle link), while maintaining perfect technique.
2. You need to continually find new ways to motivate and challenge yourself in all the exercise areas, keeping the intensity levels in your workouts high. Eventually, you may want to start adding weight resistance to your three-minute routine.
3. Don't overtrain and/or become too self-critical. This takes the joy out of working out. Incorporate transition periods into your schedule (see page 85).

STARTING THE PROGRAM

3-Minute Abs is designed for all fitness levels. Each routine has a slightly different structure. Starting out will require some trial and error to figure out how long you can exercise before resting and how much rest you need in the three-minute limit. The exercises are broken down into time units, creating flexibility within each unit. On average, each rep will take about two seconds. This means in a 30-second period you can do approximately 15 to 20 reps. The guidelines and the examples should clarify your questions.

THE IDEAL WORKOUT

The following is a template or outline of an ideal ab workout.

1. Warm-up.
2. Preparation of the neck and lower back with a few stretches.

3. A round of controlled breathing to get focused.
4. Visualization: snapshot of the abs you want to work (in your mind's eye).
5. Power phrase to get psyched up.
6. Keeping the mind-muscle link throughout the workout.
7. Cool down: controlled breathing to center your body.
8. Visualization: holding the ideal snapshot in your mind for a moment.
9. Shake it out, let it all go, and move on.

CHAPTER 8

The Program

DAY ONE LOWER-AB GUIDELINES

This routine has three rounds. Its purpose is to shape and tone your lower abdominals.

The Prescription

The ultimate goal of this routine is to do the entire routine without resting. This will, of course, depend on your fitness level. The following are examples of how different fitness levels might approach the routine.

Beginner: You may not be able to complete a round without resting. Do what you can in the allotted three-minute period. Don't get frustrated; your body will get stronger.

Intermediate: As an intermediate you may just have to rest between rounds. In the beginning you may only be able to do two rounds in the three-minute period. The goal is to work your way up to all three rounds, cutting down your rest times as you are ready.

Advanced: At this level you should be able to go through all three rounds with a minimum rest between sets, just a few seconds. As you progress at this level, you can also begin to add light weights, use a slant board, and vary the speed of repetitions.

THE ROUTINE

Detailed descriptions of the exercises follow.

Round One	Approximate Reps
Hip-ups: 30 seconds	15–20
Reverse Crunches: 30 seconds	15–20
Round Two	
Hip-ups: 30 seconds	15–20
Reverse Crunches: 30 seconds	15–20
Round Three	
Hip-ups: 30 seconds	15–20
Reverse Crunches: 30 seconds	15–20

EXERCISE Hip Raises

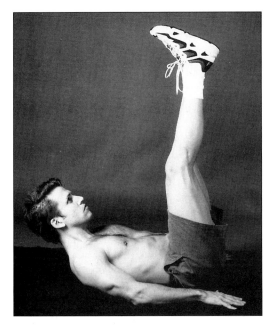
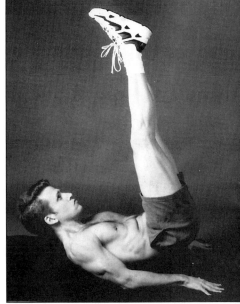

READY POSITION:

Lie flat on your back with your legs extended directly over hips (knees slightly bent). Place your hands at your sides, palms down, relax your head and neck.

THE MOTION:

Use your lower abs to elevate your hips off the floor, moving your feet straight up toward the ceiling. Then lower yourself back down in a controlled motion until your hips lightly touch the floor. Repeat.

FINE-TUNING:

- Don't kick with the legs to help elevate the hips; make lower abs do the work.
- Use your hands for stability, not to press your hips upward.
- Hold a contraction at the top of the movement.
- Focus your mind on feeling your abs do the work.
- Keep your head and neck relaxed.
- Don't rock back on upper back and neck.

EXERCISE Reverse Crunches

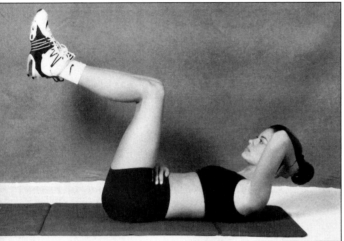

READY POSITION:
Lie flat on your back with your head and neck relaxed. Raise your thighs perpendicular to your upper body, placing your lower legs parallel to the floor.

THE MOTION:
Use your lower abs to curl your hips off the floor toward your rib cage. Lower your hips in a controlled motion until your hips touch the floor. Repeat.

Variation: Place one hand behind your head and the other hand on your lower abs so you can feel the muscle work.

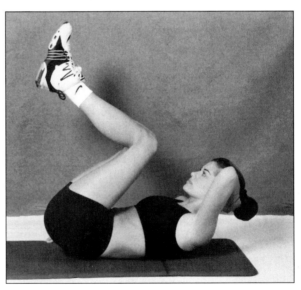

FINE-TUNING:
- Make sure the lower abs are doing the work. Don't rock, using momentum.
- Make sure you return only to the starting position. Don't rest your hips on the floor at the bottom of the movement.
- Keep constant tension on the abs.
- Focus your mind on feeling your lower abs do the work.
- Use your hands for balance. Don't use them to push off.
- Keep your neck and head relaxed.
- Don't rock back on upper back and neck.

DAY TWO **OBLIQUES**

This routine has three rounds. The goal of the routine is to trim and define your obliques so they frame and highlight your rectus abdominis. You don't want to add very much size to this area. Extra muscle mass can look like fat. And if you get too bulky, it will give you a boxy appearance instead of a nice, tapered V or curvy shape.

The Prescription

Like the other routines, your ultimate goal is to complete the routine without rest. This will, of course, depend on your fitness level. The following are examples of how different fitness levels might approach this routine.

Beginner: You may have to rest for ten or fifteen seconds after each exercise. In the beginning, you may not be able to finish round one in the three-minute period. Don't worry; increase to rounds two and three, and keep cutting down your rest times when your body is ready.

Intermediate: As an intermediate you may just have to rest between rounds. In the beginning you may be able to do only two rounds in the three-minute period. The goal is to do all three rounds without resting.

Advanced: At this level you should be able to go through all three rounds with a minimum rest between rounds, just a few seconds. As you progress you can also add weight, use a slant board, and use varying speeds of repetitions.

THE ROUTINE

Detailed descriptions of the exercises follow.

Round One
Raised Side Bends with a Cross: 30 seconds each side = 60 seconds
(approximately 15 reps each side)

Round Two
Cross Overs: 30 seconds each side = 60 seconds
(15 to 20 reps each side)

Round Three
Catches: 60 seconds
(15 to 20 reps each side)

EXERCISE Raised Side Bend with a Cross

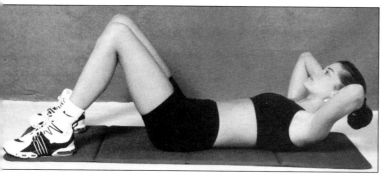

READY POSITION:
Lie on your back, knees up, feet flat on the floor, head and neck relaxed.

THE MOTION:

Raise your shoulder blades slightly off the floor, then bend at the waist, moving to your right, laterally above the floor, bringing the side of your right rib cage toward the side of your right hip. When you've moved in that direction as far as you can, raise your torso and cross your left shoulder toward your right knee. In a fluid motion, repeat this movement to the other side by lowering your left shoulder back to its original position and

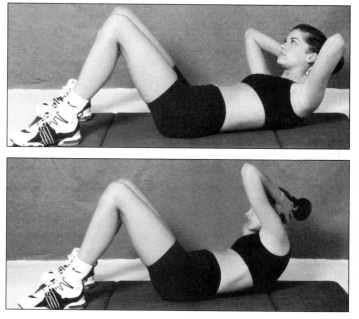

sliding your shoulder blades, still slightly raised, as far as you can to the left, then cross your right shoulder to your left knee. Be sure you keep your shoulder blades off the floor for the entire thirty-second training interval.

FINE-TUNING:

- The movement from side to side is the same as a standing side bend, except you are horizontal.
- You raise your body to place tension on the abs and allow you to move side to side.
- Move as far to the left and right as your flexibility will allow.
- Keep your shoulder blades slightly raised for the entire thirty seconds. Rest as needed.
- The crossing movement is small; you raise your torso an inch or so as it crosses diagonally

EXERCISE Cross Over

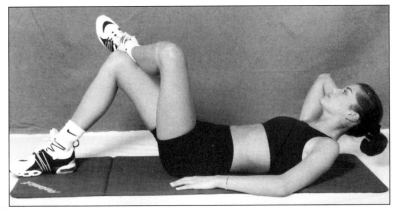

READY POSITION:
Lie on your back, knees up and both feet on the floor. Then cross your left leg over the right leg. Your left ankle should rest just below your right knee, making a triangle between your legs. Your right hand goes behind your head, elbow extended.

THE MOTION:
Use your abs to raise and cross your right shoulder toward your opposite knee. Then lower your torso back to the floor. Repeat. Reverse the procedure for the other side.
Variation: Put the hand that isn't supporting your head across your abs on the opposite oblique so you can feel the muscle work.

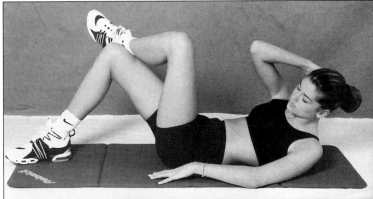

FINE-TUNING:
- Make sure your entire torso twists toward your knee. Don't just move the elbow. And don't move your knee.
- Focus your mind on feeling your obliques do the work.
- Don't rest at the bottom of the movement; keep constant tension on the abs. Hold a contraction at the top of the movement.
- Keep your head and neck relaxed.
- Keep the small of your back pressed against the floor and maintain a stable position. Do not rock.

EXERCISE Catches

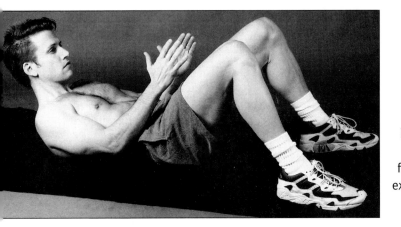

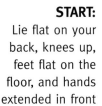

START:
Lie flat on your back, knees up, feet flat on the floor, and hands extended in front of your torso.

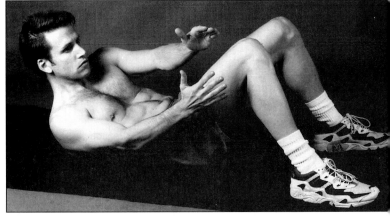

MOVEMENT:
Use your ab muscles to cross your torso on a straight, diagonal line, bringing your right shoulder toward your left knee, reaching above your left knee with both hands as if you were going to catch a ball. Lower your body back to the starting position. Repeat the movement to the opposite side.

FINE TUNING:
- Hold a contraction at the top of the movement.
- Keep constant tension on the abs. Don't rest at the bottom of the movement.
- Focus your mind on feeling the abs do the work.
- If this hurts your neck, support your neck with your hands. But still look over the top of your knee with each rep.

DAY THREE **UPPER ABS**

The goal of this routine is to bring out the definition in your upper abs. To accomplish this, crunches are done in a variety of positions, attacking this area from a variety of angles.

The Prescription

The ultimate goal of this routine is to do the entire routine without resting. This will, of course, depend on your fitness level. The following are examples of how different fitness levels might approach this routine.

Beginner: You may have to rest for ten or fifteen seconds after each exercise. In the beginning, you may be able to finish only round one in the three-minute period. Don't worry; increase to rounds two and three, and keep cutting down your rest times when your body is ready.

Intermediate: As an intermediate you may just have to rest between rounds. In the beginning, you may only be able to do two rounds in the three-minute period. The goal is to work your way up to all three rounds, cutting down your rest times as you are ready.

Advanced: At this level you should be able to go through all three rounds with a minimum rest between sets, just a few seconds. As you progress on this level you can also begin to add light weights, use a slant board, and vary the speed of repetitions.

THE ROUTINE

Detailed descriptions of the exercises follow.

Round One	Approximate Reps
Crunches: Legs Up: 30 seconds	15–20
Crunches: Knees Up: 30 seconds	15–20

Round Two	
Crunches: Feet Flat: 30 seconds	15–20
Crunches: Frogs: 30 seconds	15–20

Round Three	
Riding the Horse: 30 seconds	15–20
Crunches: Legs Up: 30 seconds	15–20

EXERCISE Crunches: Legs Up

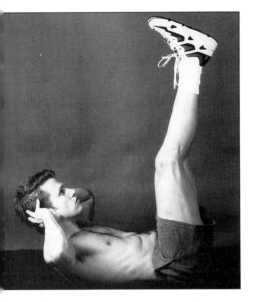 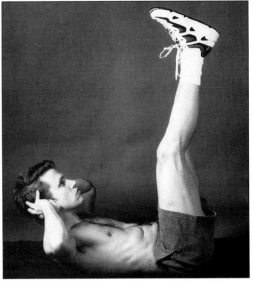

READY POSITION:
Lie flat on your back, legs straight up, perpendicular to your body (knees unlocked), head and neck relaxed.

THE MOTION:
Use your upper abs to raise your torso toward your toes, bringing your shoulder blades off the mat. Then lower your torso back to the mat. Repeat.

FINE-TUNING:
- Focus your mind on feeling the upper abs do the work.
- Don't rest at the bottom of the movement. When you feel your shoulders touch, start the next repetition.
- Hold a contraction at the top of the movement.
- If you have problems getting your legs perpendicular, sit against the wall.
- Keep your head and neck relaxed.

EXERCISE Crunches: Knees Up

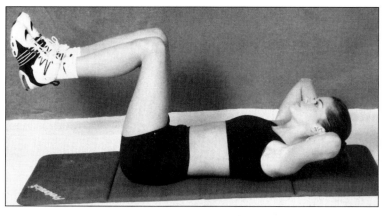

READY POSITION:
Lie on your back,
raise your legs so
your thighs are
perpendicular to your
body, placing your
lower legs parallel to
the floor, head and
neck relaxed.

THE MOTION:

Use the muscles of your upper
abs to raise your shoulders
and back off the floor in a
forward curling motion, while
crossing your right shoulder to
your left knee. Then lower
your torso to the starting
position, lightly touching your
shoulder blades to the floor.
Repeat to the other side.

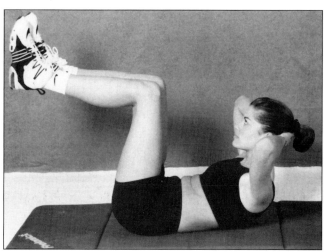

FINE-TUNING:

- Get your shoulders off the floor with each repetition; don't just move your neck up and down.
- Keep the movement controlled.
- Hold a contraction at the top of each movement.
- Don't rest your shoulders on the floor at the bottom of the movement.
- Focus your mind on feeling your upper abs do the work.
- Keep your head and neck relaxed.

EXERCISE Crunches: Knees Bent

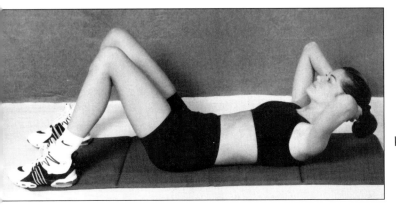

READY POSITION:
Lie on your back, knees bent, so your feet rest flat on the floor, neck and head relaxed.

THE MOTION:
Use your upper abs to raise your shoulder blades off the floor in a forward curling motion. Then lower your shoulders to the starting position, lightly touching your shoulder blades to the floor. Repeat.

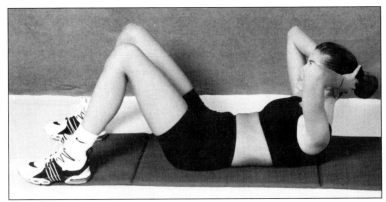

FINE-TUNING:
- Keep constant tension on your abs throughout the movement.
- Focus your mind on feeling your upper abs do the work.
- Don't rest at the bottom of the movement.
- Hold a contraction at the top of the movement.
- Make sure you move your shoulders off the floor. Don't just move your neck and head.
- Keep the small of your back pressed against the floor.
- Keep your head and neck relaxed.

EXERCISE Crunches: Frog Legs

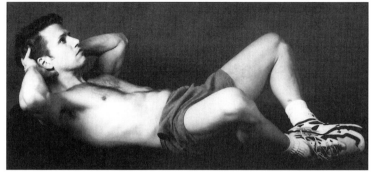

READY POSITION:
Lie on your back, bring the soles of your feet together, keeping your feet on the ground, head and neck relaxed.

THE MOTION:
Using the muscles of your upper abs, raise your shoulder blades off the floor in a curling motion. Then lower your shoulders to starting position, lightly touching the floor. Repeat.

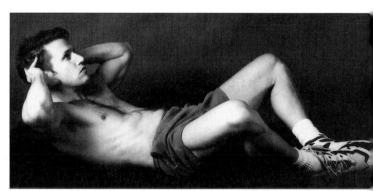

FINE-TUNING:
- Keep constant tension on your abs.
- Focus your mind on your upper abs, feeling them do the work.
- Don't rest at the bottom of the movement.
- Hold a contraction at the top of the movement.
- Make sure you move your shoulders off the floor. Don't just move your neck and head.
- Keep your lower back pressed against the floor.
- Keep your neck and head relaxed.

EXERCISE Crunches: Riding the Horse

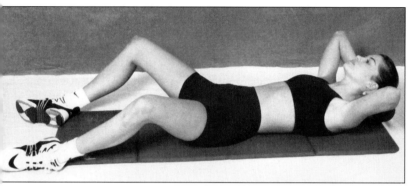

READY POSITION:
Lie on your back,
extend and round
your legs like you
are riding a horse,
head and neck
relaxed.

THE MOTION:
Using the muscles
of your upper abs,
raise your shoulder
blades off the floor
in a curling motion.
Then lower your
shoulders to
starting position,
lightly touching the
floor. Repeat.

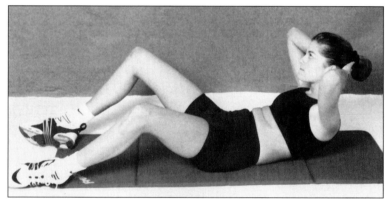

FINE-TUNING:
- Keep constant tension on your abs.
- Focus your mind on your upper abs, feeling them do the work.
- Don't rest at the bottom of the movement.
- Hold a contraction at the top of the movement.
- Make sure you move your shoulders off the floor. Don't just move your neck and head.
- Keep your lower back pressed against the floor.
- Keep your neck and head relaxed.

CHAPTER 9

3-Minute Wellness

The big picture means looking at yourself holistically. Besides the physical element of wellness, which is the primary focus of this book, there are five other categories. The following section is a brief overview of these categories.

PHYSICAL DEVELOPMENT is the care of your physical body. This includes your daily exercise program, eating healthy, personal hygiene, and medical care. This also means not abusing tobacco, drugs, and alcohol, getting enough sleep, wearing seat belts, etc.

EMOTIONAL DEVELOPMENT emphasizes awareness and acceptance of one's feelings and finding constructive ways to use these emotions. The emotionally well person maintains satisfying relationships with others while feeling positive and enthusiastic about his/her own life.

INTELLECTUAL DEVELOPMENT encourages creative and open-minded mental activities. Active involvement in literature and the arts are two prime examples. The intellectually well person takes responsibility for continuing his/her intellectual development.

SOCIAL DEVELOPMENT relates to your community and physical environment. A socially well person emphasizes interdependence with his or her environment and pursues harmony with family, friends, and associates. This person has developed healthy ways to interact, react, and live with all types of people.

VOCATIONAL DEVELOPMENT encourages the pursuit and growth of one's attitude towards his/her work. A vocationally well person seeks jobs that bring personal satisfaction and enrichment into his/her life.

SPIRITUAL DEVELOPMENT involves seeking meaning and purpose in human existence. A spiritually well person forms a strong appreciation for the experience of being alive.

HOW THE DIMENSIONS AFFECT US

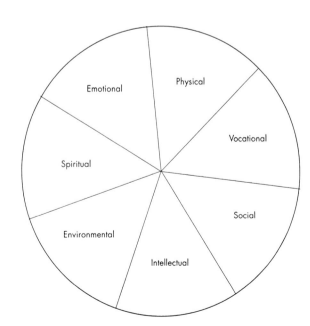

An easy way to see how these dimensions interrelate is to look at the whole picture as a pie chart. Each piece represents a dimension of wellness. A problem within one piece affects the whole pie.

For example, if you recently fell and broke your ankle, your physical wellness has been taxed. Because of this, it is likely that vocational wellness may suffer if your job requires you to be active and you miss work. You would also be emotionally stressed, not to mention the social impact of an injury on family and friends. All the dimensions intermingle, creating your web of wellness.

It's important to understand that every pie chart will be different. For instance, a professor at a university may have a larger piece of pie for the intellectual dimension than an athlete, whose physical dimension would be larger. Your pie chart will reflect your individuality.

THE PHYSICAL DIMENSION: OVERVIEW

Because this is a fitness book, let's take a closer look at the physical piece of the pie, specifically exercise.

The four ELEMENTS of exercise wellness are cardiovascular exercise, muscular strengthening and endurance, flexibility, and nutrition/diet (see chapter 12). To have a well-rounded physical wellness profile you need to include each of these four elements in your exercise program.

CARDIOVASCULAR

Activities that tax the heart, lungs, and circulatory systems improve cardiovascular fitness. Cardiovascular exercise puts a demand on the oxygen exchange systems of your body. Oxygen has to be taken in from the lungs to the circulatory system, then distributed to the muscles that are being used during exercise. The oxygen is utilized to convert fats into energy. This entire exchange system forces the lungs and heart to become extremely efficient during exercise, so that the working muscles can continue their activities.

The American College of Sports Medicine states that thirty

minutes of cardiovascular exercise at least three times a week is sufficient to receive health benefits. A cardiovascular program consists of activities that allow you to reach 65–85 percent of your maximum heart rate for a duration of at least twenty minutes.

STRENGTH TRAINING

Weight training increases the strength and endurance of your muscles. Other benefits include better posture, stronger bones and ligaments, increased muscle tone and flexibility, and improved strength in your joints.

Strength training should include exercises designed for all major muscle groups of the body. The exercises should be performed at least two to three times per week. Strength training can be done in a variety of ways: free weights, machines, or body weight.

You should not begin a strength program without help from a qualified trainer. Learning proper technique from the beginning ensures a safe and effective training program.

FLEXIBILITY

Flexibility is usually the most neglected element of a training program. Flexibility training works the muscles, ligaments, and joints. Stretching is important for the maintenance of posture, joint mobility, and range of motion. Flexibility training needs to be done at least three times a week and should provide stretches for all major muscle groups and joints.

THE CHALLENGE

The challenge of three-minute wellness is simple, so simple we forget to do it. Wellness is an exercise in awareness. Once a week challenge yourself to spend three minutes meditating on the big picture, the six areas of wellness, and choose one action that will bring greater balance into your life. It can be as simple as reading the arts page in the paper or giving your mother a call. It sounds simple, right? Give it a try and week by week see how your life changes.

CHAPTER 10

The 3-Minute Stretch

THE STRETCHING PROGRAM

The following routine stretches the key muscles involved in ab work.

Neck Stretch: Each stretch should be done once; then move on to the next movement without resting.

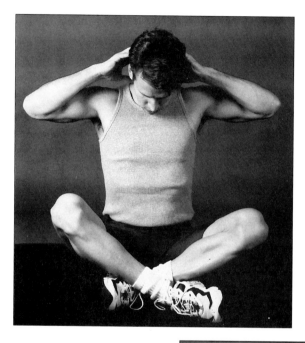

Drop head forward, chin to chest. Hold for ten seconds.

Looking straight ahead, lower your ear to your shoulder. Hold for ten seconds. Lower your other ear to your other shoulder. Hold for ten seconds.

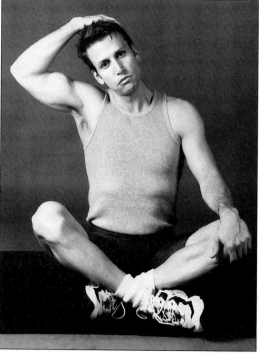

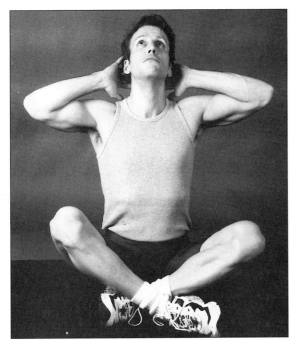

Then gently extend your neck backwards, using your hands for support. Hold for ten seconds.

Knees-to-Chest Hug: Lie flat on your back, bringing both knees to your chest. From this position, wrap your arms around your legs and hug your knees to your chest. At the same time, bring your chin to your chest. Hold for fifteen seconds.

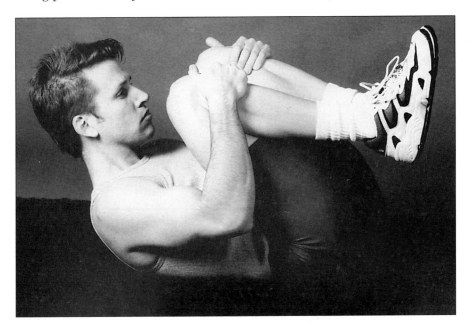

Knees to Side: Lie flat on your back, knees bent, feet flat on the floor. Let both legs fall to one side. Hold for ten seconds. Then let the legs fall to the other side. Hold for ten seconds.

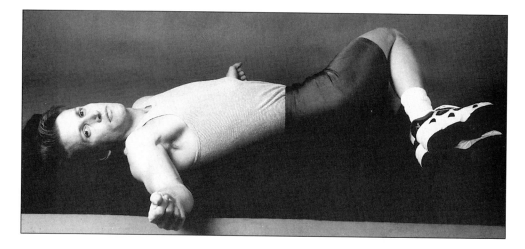

Back Stretch: Lie on your stomach, hands under your chest (palms down). Pressing up with your arms, slowly raise your torso and head while keeping your hips on the ground. Keep your lower body relaxed. Hold for fifteen seconds; lower torso back to starting position.

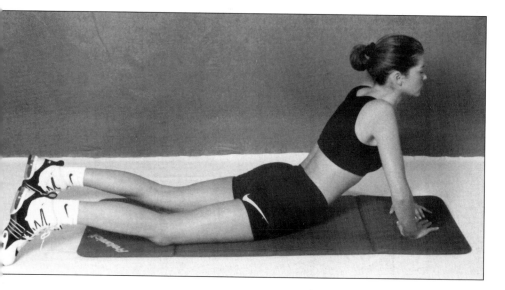

Back Arch: Come up on your hands and knees (all fours). Place your hands under your shoulders and round your back up like a cat, lowering your head. Hold for ten seconds and perform two reps.

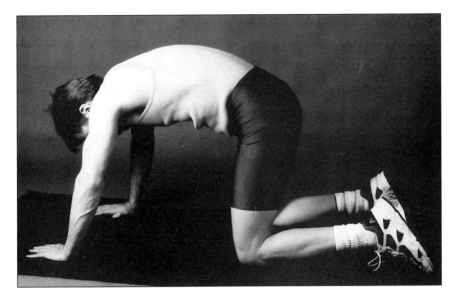

Then arch your back in the opposite direction, raising your head. Hold for ten seconds.

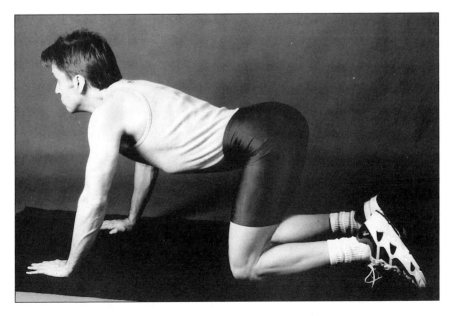

CHAPTER 11

Lower Back

Strengthening the Weak Link

LOWER BACK AND THE ABS

The abdominals play a central role in the prevention and rehabilitation of lower-back pain. The abs and the lower back are partners. Imagine the torso as a large barrel wrapped with steel bands for support, and inside the barrel are your body's essential organs. The abdominal muscles act like these steel bands, supporting and stabilizing the torso. Weak abdominal muscles allow the stomach to sag, increasing the load on the lower back: your lumbar extensors, vertebrae, and discs.

THE UNGUARDED MOMENT

Most lower-back injuries occur during an "unguarded moment," when you have to suddenly react to a change in the environment. It can occur when one turns, twists, stoops, or bends in an unusual manner. Strengthening your lower back makes it able to withstand greater external loads and decreases injury rates.

ACUTE AND CHRONIC PAIN

When back pain continues beyond six weeks, it is considered chronic. An individual suffering from chronic low-back pain will subconsciously learn new muscle recruitment patterns that substitute for a weak and painful low back. This is a primitive neuromotor survival strategy that allowed our ancestors to escape danger even in the event of injury. The natural reaction to back pain is to splint or guard any movements that require the back to work. This temporarily shields the back muscles from exposure to external forces and relieves short-term pain. But the long-term effects can be devastating. Pain leads to disuse; disuse leads to muscular atrophy; atrophy leads to weakness. Weakness makes you vulnerable to injury. This continuous cycle is referred to as the *chronic deconditioning syndrome*. Chronic deconditioning syndrome is like having a cast on your arm. After removal of the cast, the muscles in the arm are weaker. The human body physiologically adapts to the demands placed upon it. The muscle group in question has essentially adapted to no stimulation, becoming weak.

You can increase a muscle's strength by exposing it to regular overload stimulation (strength training). In other words, by isolating and strengthening the muscles, you can treat and prevent back pain. Increasing your levels of strength increases your structural integrity and your ability to withstand the unguarded moment. Specific exercise is the only effective way to prevent lower-back problems. It is also the only effective way to rehabilitate and control the recurrence of chronic lower-back pain once it has developed.

BASIC GUIDELINES FOR BACK STRENGTHENING

The following exercises will help you strengthen the muscles of your lower back. They are listed in order of difficulty.

- Always work within a comfortable range of motion in which you feel no pain.
- Stop the movement just prior to the point of discomfort. Resistance training strengthens the muscle beyond the range of motion.
- Never use a sudden movement when performing a strength exercise.
- By performing a slow, controlled movement, you will not be able to handle as much resistance, but muscular fatigue (overload) is still accomplished, and the risk of injury is reduced.

Opposite Arm and Leg: On Knees

READY POSITION:
Start on all fours, resting on your hands and knees.

THE MOTION:
Simultaneously raise and straighten your right arm and left leg until they are parallel to the ground (or as close to parallel as you can without going past the parallel position).

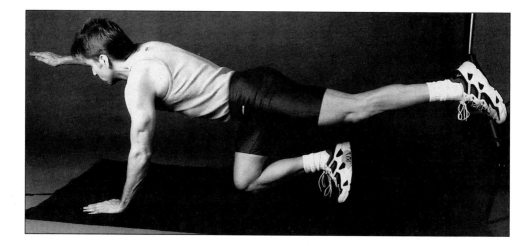

PRESCRIPTION:
Hold for two seconds and come back slowly to the starting position. Start with ten repetitions on each side and build up to twenty repetitions. Repeat with left arm and right leg.

Opposite Arm and Leg on Stomach: Facedown

READY POSITION:
Lie facedown on the floor, arms extended overhead, palms on the floor.

THE MOTION:
Simultaneously raise your right arm and left leg to a comfortable height.

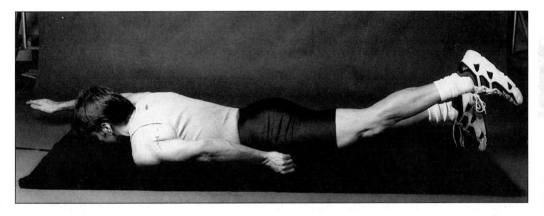

PRESCRIPTION:
Hold for two seconds and come back to the floor slowly. Build up to twenty repetitions. Repeat with left arm and right leg.

Basic
Back Extension

READY POSITION:

Lie facedown, flat on the floor. Place your heels under a support
(a couch or have a partner hold your ankles down), arms at your sides.
It is also possible to do this exercise without leg support.

THE MOTION:

Slowly raise your chest off the floor as high as you can.

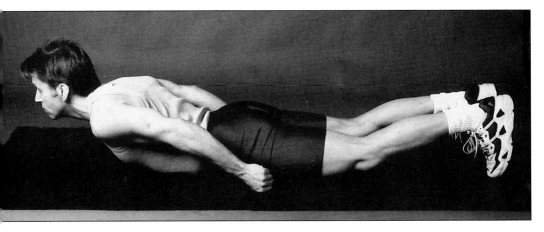

PRESCRIPTION:

Hold for two seconds and come back to the floor slowly. Gradually
increase until you can do twenty repetitions easily.

Intermediate
Back Extension

READY POSITION:

Lie facedown with a firm pillow under your pelvis. Place your heels under a support (a couch or have a partner hold your ankles down), arms to your sides.

THE MOTION:

Slowly, raise your chest off the floor to a comfortable height.

PRESCRIPTION:

Hold for two seconds and come back to the floor slowly. When you can do twenty repetitions easily, place another pillow under your pelvis. This will increase the difficulty and range of motion of the exercise. (This exercise is the same as Basic Back Extension, except that you place a pillow under your hips.)

FOR THOSE WITH LOWER-BACK PROBLEMS

If you have lower-back problems, you face special challenges when working out. It is important for you to start slowly and build gradually. You may feel that you can do more during the early phases, but remember it is quality, not quantity. You need to be careful and gradually develop a foundation of strength. Your lower-back problems didn't develop overnight, and restoration of function won't either.

When exercising, it is also important that you learn how to distinguish between good and bad pain, as discussed earlier. If you have a history of lower-back pain, you should *not* exercise through spasm, lingering pain, or shooting, peripheral pain. And remember, it is always imperative that you check with a doctor before beginning an exercise program.

The important thing to remember is, if you have a lower-back problem, part of the problem is lower-back weakness. You have to strengthen the weak area. Proper stretching and specific lower-back exercises will help strengthen and prevent recurring back pain. If you take care of your back, it will last a lifetime, but strength and movement are the keys.

CHAPTER 12

3-Minute Diet Guide

(or the Top Ten Tips)

If you have been working out, but have not been getting the results you expected, the reason is probably connected to what you eat. Food choices are the fuel for fitness and play a major role in body fat composition. The type of fuel that you put in your body affects your performance. So, if you want your workouts to pay off, eat for energy and power. Here are ten steps you can begin today.

1. Eating at least two servings of fruits and vegetables at every meal. That means about one cup cooked (including canned) or two cups raw. Use some juice if you like, but eat mostly whole fruits and vegetables. Fruits and vegetables are full of antioxidants, fiber, and other nutrients that can't be replaced with a vitamin pill or sport supplement. They are low in calories but packed with nutrition.

A day's worth of these power-packed foods might look like this: A six-ounce glass of orange juice and two small bananas on whole-grain cereal for breakfast. Two or three thick tomato slices and several fresh spinach leaves on your sandwich at lunch. Add low-fat cole slaw or a fresh peach as your second serving. For dinner, have a small baked potato and half a cup of steamed carrots or broccoli with your entrée. Now, that's not so hard.

2. Eat protein at every meal. People tend to feel more energetic throughout the day when eating protein at every meal instead of one big serving at dinner. Think in terms of having small to moderate servings—yogurt at breakfast, tuna at lunch, low-fat cheese as a snack, and beans for dinner, for example.

How much protein is enough? If you are weight training or doing endurance sports training, shoot for one gram of protein per pound of body weight. You will need only half that amount if you are exercising at a moderate level without weights. You will likely get enough protein if half to two-thirds of your daily requirement comes from protein-dense foods such as yogurt, skim milk or soy milk, nonfat or low-fat cheese, lean meats, fish and seafood, beans, peas, and tofu. Look for the protein content of foods on the nutrition facts food label.

3. Eat mostly healthy fats to meet your essential fatty acid needs. Most active adults can eat up to about sixty fat grams a day and still have a "low-fat" diet. Cutting fat intake too much, below thirty fat grams a day, can cause fatigue, a compromised immune system, dry skin, excess hunger, and an unbalanced diet high in sugar and fat-free junk foods.

Don't be afraid of healthy fats—oils, nuts, seeds, avocado, olives, nut butters, salmon, flaxseeds or oil, and wheat germ. Cook in small amounts of oil instead of butter, margarine, or shortening. Add a few almonds to salads. Have avocado slices on your sandwich. Dip raw carrots and celery in almond or natural peanut butter. Use nonfat dairy products and lean meats.

4. Eat several times a day. Skipping meals leads to overeating. Remember, your body is burning calories all day long and needs to be refueled every four to six hours. This keeps you feeling energetic and keeps your metabolism revved up.

Don't kid yourself into thinking coffee and a doughnut constitute a meal. Caffeine and sugar will keep you hyped up for a while, but you need real food for real energy. With a little planning, it takes only a few minutes longer to eat a healthy meal than a junk snack.

5. Make complex carbohydrates your primary fuel source. This includes vegetables and whole grains. Instead of living on white flour products, such as bagels, pretzels, and pasta, try eating more whole-wheat toast, brown and wild rice, oatmeal, and other whole grains. Whole grains will add fiber, small amounts of essential fats, and more vitamins and minerals to your diet. At least half of all the grain, flour, cereal, and bread products you eat need to be whole grain. By the way, "wheat" does not mean "whole wheat," so read your food labels!

6. Go easy on the alcohol and caffeine. Both are dehydrating, which will zap energy for workouts. If you drink more than two cups of coffee or tea and more than one serving of alcohol a day, cut back. Once you get used to less caffeine and alcohol, you will feel more energized and your workouts will be more productive.

7. Drink eight to ten glasses of water a day. Staying well hydrated is essential to nutritional fitness. You can count milk, juice, and soup as part of your daily fluid requirement, but water is your best bet for hydrating your body.

8. Listen to your body cues. Let your body tell you how much to eat. Children do this naturally, but adults tend to override their internal cues by eating when it's convenient. Your body has a built-in calorie control mechanism that works pretty well, especially if you are active and eating mostly healthy foods. Eat when physically hungry and stop when you have reached that "just right" feeling of satiety. If you don't know what I am talking about, then you are probably out of touch with your body's hunger cues. It's time to slow down and listen.

Before you take that first bite, ask yourself, "Am I hungry?" If the answer is yes, then eat. If the answer is no, wait. After eating about half your meal, ask "Do I need more to feel physically satisfied?" Stop eating when your body answers "no" to that question.

9. Put your body weight into a healthy perspective. Fitness is more important than leanness. If your goal is to have well-toned muscles (the abdominal six-pack), then you have to be very lean: 8 to 10 percent body fat for men, 15 to 18 eighteen percent body fat for women. Is this a body you can live in comfortably, without obsessing about every fat gram you eat and every ounce you weigh? If this is too rigorous, focus on eating for energy and health and let the pounds fall where they may. Everyone will have a different answer to this question. For some people the answer will change from season to season.

10. If in doubt, take a balanced vitamin and mineral supplement daily. In today's world, most people do not take the time to eat well. Plus, nutrition research suggests there may be good reasons to supplement our diets with certain nutrients for disease prevention. It is usually safe to take a multiple vitamin/mineral supplement that contains 100 percent of the U.S. RDA (recommended daily allowance) for nutrients. Additional levels of specific nutrients, such as vitamin E, vitamin C, and calcium, may be wise, depending on your diet and health status. After getting your diet in order, consult with a qualified nutritionist about taking supplements. If you are under medical supervision or taking medication, consult your physician before taking nutritional supplements.

CHAPTER 13

Gender and Abs

A 3-Minute Tour

Your gender is the single biggest factor that defines your physical body. There is no value judgment in this. Each gender has its strengths and weaknesses.

This chapter will outline the basic differences that are important for your ab training.

As you look at the following pages, remember this old piece of advice:

Accept the things you cannot change, change the things you can, and have the wisdom to know the difference.

THE MAN

- The average man has between 14 and 18 percent body fat. This is less than women have. It is easier for a man to get muscular definition.
- But men are predisposed to store fat on their obliques (love handles). It is the first place men put on weight and the last place they take it off. So it is hard to get rid of that extra inch without starving yourself.
- It is easier for a man to gain muscle because he has higher levels of testosterone in his body. This makes it easier for a man to develop his rectus abdominis muscle, creating the "washboard abs" look.
- And a man's abs cover more area than a woman's. (Women have smaller waists and bigger hips.) This makes the abs a very visible part of the male body.
- But this extra area and greater potential for muscle growth can make the abs look fatter if your body fat percentage is high.

THE WOMAN

- The average woman has between 20 and 24 percent body fat. The good news (abwise) is this gets stored primarily in the butt and thighs.
- However, women have a tendency to also store fat in their lower abs, below the belly button, commonly called "the pooch." This area is at approximately the same level as the hips.
- Because women have a naturally higher body fat percentage, it is also more difficult for them to get the same definition as a man. A woman would have to go on an extremely low-calorie diet to get "cut up" like a man.
- Women also have lower levels of testosterone in their bodies, so it is harder for them to develop ab muscles that "pop" like a man's. In other words, it is very difficult for a woman to get washboard abs. But this lack of muscular mass creates a small and curvaceous midriff.
- After pregnancy it is hard for a woman to get prepregnancy tightness back in her abs. Hormones have caused the collagen tissue to relax and stretch to aid childbirth. The abs can still be tightened and toned, but they may not return to prepregnancy form.

CHAPTER 14

The Long Haul

As you continue your fitness journey, you're going to learn more about training and your body—your strengths and weaknesses. You will start to have little dialogues with your body. You will get better at both asking questions and listening. Your training will become more intuitive. To help you in this process, this chapter discusses the two basic training stages: peaking out, and transition or rest periods.

PERIODIZATION

Periodization is a systematic and progressive training method designed to aid in planning and organization. This chapter will be a brief overview of this system. It will give you the broad strokes to superimpose on your training program.

YOU'VE GOT TO ADAPT

The basis for periodization is derived from the General Adaptation Syndrome (GAS), which was developed during the 1930s. It was intended to describe a person's ability to adapt to stress. There are three distinct phases to the GAS:[1]

1. *Alarm Stage*—This relates to the individual's initial response to training. This could manifest itself as a temporary drop in performance due to stiffness or soreness.
2. *Resistance Stage*—In this stage the individual adapts to the training stimulus by making certain adjustments. These adjustments may include physiological (training techniques) and psychological adaptations. The adaptations in this stage are positive, leading you to your desired result.
3. *Exhaustion or Overwork Stage*—When the total stress placed upon the individual is too great, signs of overtraining manifest themselves:

   A loss of strength or plateauing of performance.
   Chronic fatigue.
   Loss of appetite.
   Loss of body weight, or lean body mass.
   Illness.
   Injury.
   Decreased motivation and low self-esteem.

   In the exhaustion stage, you will not make the desired training adaptations. Outside stress—social life, improper nutrition, lack of sleep, long work hours—also need to be considered to avoid overtraining.

The goal is to remain in the resistance stage of training (number two), with periodic moves into the alarm stage. This allows your body to adapt to stresses while continually improving. Being aware of these cycles will help keep your training program on the right track.

THE PEAKING PERIOD

All your training ELEMENTS culminate in this period. This will, of course, be different for everybody. For the elite athlete, this can be very complicated, because several variables have to come together at once: strength, endurance, specific sports skills, diet, mental state, etc. The same is true for a bodybuilder.

If you want your abs to reach a peak for a vacation on the beach, you should be focusing on three variables:

- Your abdominal routine.
- Diet.
- Cardiovascular training.

But your mental state is also important; you don't want to go to the beach with a bad attitude. No one will want to build sand castles with you.

TRANSITION

Unfortunately, maintaining peak anything for a long period of time can be very difficult. The stress of staying in peak condition leads to stage three, overtraining and burnout. The cycle or period of time following a peaking period must be a transition phase.

Transition is designed to introduce variety into the program while bringing about recovery and recuperation, both mentally and physically. It is good old R and R. And, as the term *transition* implies, this phase will allow you to move to a higher training level.

When most people think of recuperation they think of sitting on their butt and doing nothing. In the transition phase you will continue to engage in activities but at low volumes and intensities. These activities should be physical activities that you enjoy. Depending upon your goals for the next peaking period, the transition phase will usually last from one to two weeks.

Peaking out and transition are the two bookends of the training cycle. It is essential to remember the two lessons of these cycles: (1) you can't stay in peak condition for long periods of time (that equals burnout), and (2) the transition cycle is not about laziness; it is a necessary step for getting to the next level.

People often assume that taking time off will cause them to fall behind, when in reality it is a necessary part of moving ahead. The applications of these principles will lead to your ultimate success and longevity in training.

As you progress on your fitness journey, listen to your body and use common sense; don't believe the images the media hurls at you. *3-Minute Abs* will lead the way, showing you that a little bit of hard, consistent work goes a long way. This program is an opportunity to practice and perfect all the key elements of training, just like professional bodybuilders and athletes. Since each session is so short, it is a chance to establish good habits. In each session, commit your mind and body to staying focused, practicing perfect technique, and pushing toward your goals.

Train hard and train smart.